PRE DIABETES MEAL PLANNING COOKBOOK FOR VEGETARIANS AND VEGANS

Delicious Plant-Based Recipes and Meal Plans to Prevent and Reverse Prediabetes

By Mia Bennett

COPYRIGHT PAGE

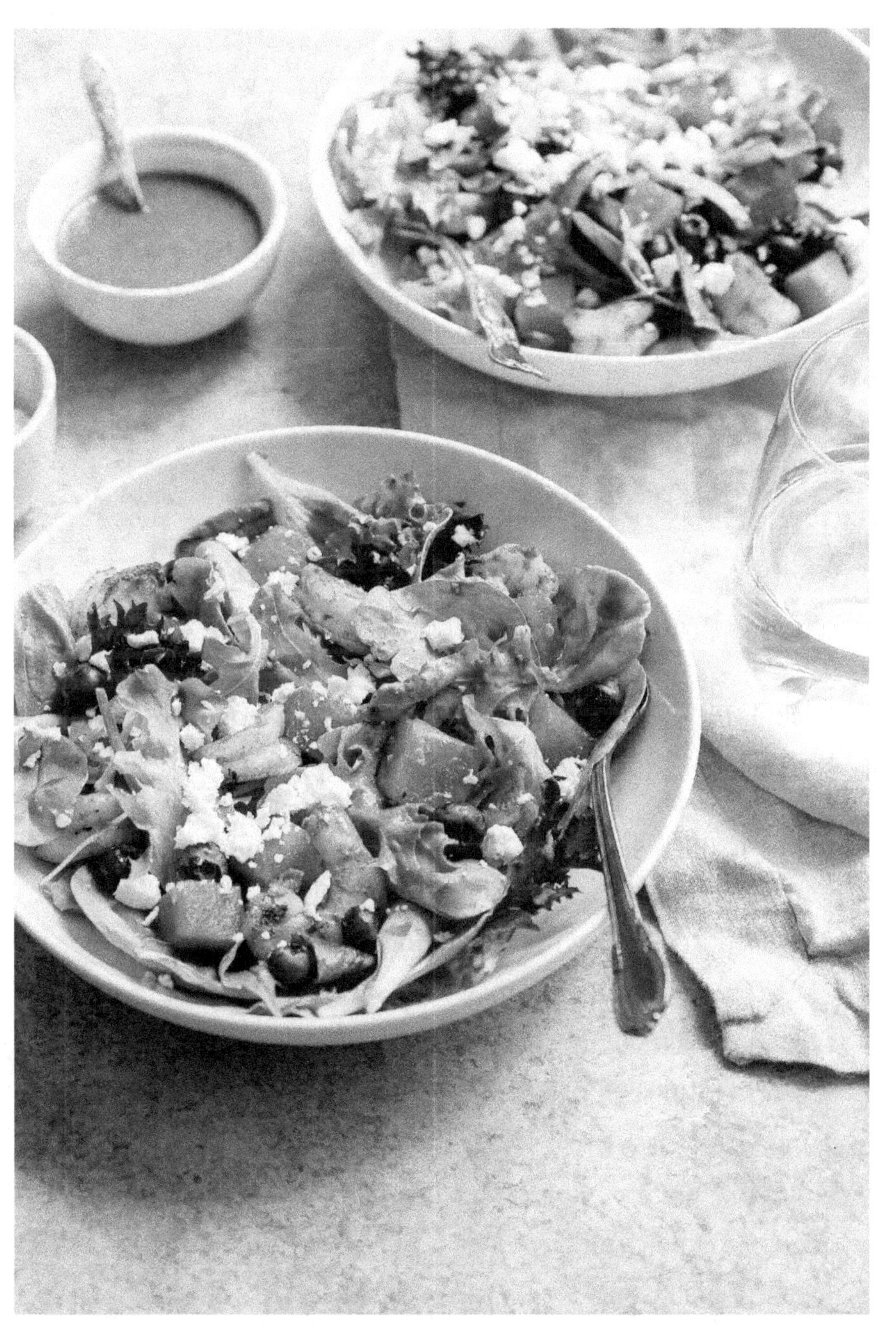

TABLE OF CONTENTS

INTRODUCTION

I magine your body's response to sugar is like a traffic jam. Normally, insulin, a hormone, acts like traffic police, ushering sugar into your cells for energy. In prediabetes, the sugar traffic gets congested – your body produces insulin, but the cells become resistant, leading to high blood sugar levels. This isn't full-blown diabetes yet, but it's a warning sign.

Here's the good news: prediabetes is a wake-up call you can answer. Diet plays a starring role in managing it, and plant-based diets like vegetarian and vegan can be powerful tools.

Understanding Prediabetes: The Body's Traffic Jam

Think of prediabetes as a crossroads. Left unchecked, it can lead to type 2 diabetes, a chronic condition affecting how your body regulates blood sugar. But with lifestyle changes, you can prevent this progression.

Several factors contribute to prediabetes, including genetics, weight, and physical activity level. Diet, however, is a modifiable risk factor you can directly address.

Diet as Your Traffic Cop: Regulating Blood Sugar Flow

Refined carbohydrates and sugary drinks are like fast lanes for sugar, causing rapid spikes in blood sugar levels. This overwhelms your insulin system, worsening the traffic jam.

A prediabetes-friendly diet focuses on whole, unprocessed foods. Here's how it works:

- **Fiber Power:** Fiber-rich vegetables, fruits, whole grains, and legumes act like stop signs, slowing down sugar absorption and preventing blood sugar spikes.
- **Nutrient Balance**: Plant-based proteins, healthy fats, and essential vitamins and minerals from whole foods support overall health and insulin sensitivity.

The Vegetarian and Vegan Advantage: A Plant-Based Path to Better Blood Sugar Control

Vegetarian and vegan diets are naturally lower in saturated fat and cholesterol, often linked to insulin resistance. They're also typically abundant in fiber, keeping your blood sugar on a smooth ride.

Studies have shown that plant-based diets can improve blood sugar control, promote weight loss (if needed), and reduce the risk of developing type 2 diabetes.

Making Plant-Based Work for You

Whether you choose lacto-ovo vegetarian (including dairy and eggs), lacto-vegetarian (dairy only), or vegan (no animal products), a well-planned plant-based diet can be highly beneficial for prediabetes management.

Here are some tips:

- **Variety is Key:** Explore the rainbow of fruits and vegetables, ensuring you get a good mix of vitamins, minerals, and antioxidants.
- **Protein Power:** Include plant-based protein sources like legumes, nuts, seeds, and whole grains to feel full and support healthy blood sugar levels.
- **Healthy Fats:** Don't shy away from healthy fats like avocados, nuts, and olive oil. They promote satiety and support nutrient absorption.

Remember: Prediabetes doesn't have to be a dead end. By taking charge of your diet, particularly with the potential benefits of plant-based approaches, you can manage your blood sugar, improve your health, and steer yourself towards a healthier future.

Chapter 1: 30-Day Meal Plan

Week 1

Day 1

- Breakfast: Oatmeal with Berries and Almonds
- Lunch: Lentil and Vegetable Soup
- Dinner: Eggplant Parmesan
- Snack: Hummus and Crudites
- Dessert: Vegan Chocolate Avocado Mousse

Day 2

- Breakfast: Tofu Scramble with Spinach and Tomatoes
- Lunch: Chickpea Salad with Lemon Dressing
- Dinner: Cauliflower Steak with Chimichurri
- Snack: Edamame with Sea Salt
- Dessert: Berry Coconut Parfait

Day 3

- Breakfast: Chia Seed Pudding with Fresh Fruit
- Lunch: Stuffed Bell Peppers with Quinoa and Black Beans
- Dinner: Vegan Chili with Quinoa
- Snack: Guacamole with Whole Grain Tortilla Chips
- Dessert: Pumpkin Pie Energy Bites

Day 4

- Breakfast: Whole Grain Pancakes with Maple Syrup
- Lunch: Vegan Caesar Salad with Tofu
- Dinner: Ratatouille with Polenta
- Snack: Stuffed Dates with Almond Butter
- Dessert: Banana Nice Cream

Day 5

- Breakfast: Avocado Toast with Chickpeas
- Lunch: Spinach and Mushroom Quesadilla
- Dinner: Mushroom and Spinach Risotto
- Snack: Roasted Chickpeas with Paprika
- Dessert: Vegan Lemon Bars

Day 6

- Breakfast: Vegan Breakfast Burrito
- Lunch: Mediterranean Couscous Salad
- Dinner: Butternut Squash Curry
- Snack: Caprese Skewers with Balsamic Glaze
- Dessert: Almond Butter Cookies

Day 7

- Breakfast: Quinoa Breakfast Bowl
- Lunch: Sweet Potato and Black Bean Tacos

- Dinner: Stuffed Acorn Squash with Wild Rice

- Snack: Vegan Spinach Artichoke Dip

- Dessert: Chia Seed Chocolate Pudding

Week 2

Day 8

- Breakfast: Fruit and Nut Granola

- Lunch: Vegan Buddha Bowl

- Dinner: Vegan Shepherd's Pie

- Snack: Sliced Apple with Nut Butter

- Dessert: Mango Sorbet

Day 9

- Breakfast: Smoothie Bowl with Greens and Berries

- Lunch: Zucchini Noodles with Pesto

- Dinner: Lemon Garlic Pasta with Asparagus

- Snack: Vegan Cheese and Crackers

- Dessert: Vegan Apple Crisp

Day 10

- Breakfast: Vegan French Toast

- Lunch: Greek Salad with Tofu Feta

- Dinner: Black Bean and Sweet Potato Enchiladas

- Snack: Quinoa and Black Bean Stuffed Mini Peppers
- Dessert: Pistachio Date Balls

Day 11

- Breakfast: Buckwheat Porridge with Cinnamon
- Lunch: Quinoa Stuffed Portobello Mushrooms
- Dinner: Vegan Pad Thai
- Snack: Coconut Yogurt with Fresh Berries
- Dessert: Blueberry Oat Bars

Day 12

- Breakfast: Almond Butter Overnight Oats
- Lunch: Thai Peanut Noodle Salad
- Dinner: Portobello Mushroom Burgers
- Snack: Trail Mix with Nuts and Seeds
- Dessert: Coconut Macaroons

Day 13

- Breakfast: Sweet Potato Hash with Kale
- Lunch: Vegan Minestrone Soup
- Dinner: Lentil Bolognese with Whole Wheat Pasta
- Snack: Veggie Sushi Rolls
- Dessert: Vegan Carrot Cake

Day 14

- Breakfast: Breakfast Quinoa with Coconut Milk
- Lunch: Falafel Wrap with Hummus
- Dinner: Moroccan Chickpea Stew
- Snack: Baked Sweet Potato Fries
- Dessert: Peanut Butter Chocolate Chip Blondies

Week 3

Day 15

- Breakfast: Oatmeal with Berries and Almonds
- Lunch: Lentil and Vegetable Soup
- Dinner: Eggplant Parmesan
- Snack: Hummus and Crudites
- Dessert: Vegan Chocolate Avocado Mousse

Day 16

- Breakfast: Tofu Scramble with Spinach and Tomatoes
- Lunch: Chickpea Salad with Lemon Dressing
- Dinner: Cauliflower Steak with Chimichurri
- Snack: Edamame with Sea Salt
- Dessert: Berry Coconut Parfait

Day 17

- Breakfast: Chia Seed Pudding with Fresh Fruit
- Lunch: Stuffed Bell Peppers with Quinoa and Black Beans
- Dinner: Vegan Chili with Quinoa
- Snack: Guacamole with Whole Grain Tortilla Chips
- Dessert: Pumpkin Pie Energy Bites

Day 18

- Breakfast: Whole Grain Pancakes with Maple Syrup
- Lunch: Vegan Caesar Salad with Tofu
- Dinner: Ratatouille with Polenta
- Snack: Stuffed Dates with Almond Butter
- Dessert: Banana Nice Cream

Day 19

- Breakfast: Avocado Toast with Chickpeas
- Lunch: Spinach and Mushroom Quesadilla
- Dinner: Mushroom and Spinach Risotto
- Snack: Roasted Chickpeas with Paprika
- Dessert: Vegan Lemon Bars

Day 20

- Breakfast: Vegan Breakfast Burrito
- Lunch: Mediterranean Couscous Salad

- Dinner: Butternut Squash Curry

- Snack: Caprese Skewers with Balsamic Glaze

- Dessert: Almond Butter Cookies

Day 21

- Breakfast: Quinoa Breakfast Bowl

- Lunch: Sweet Potato and Black Bean Tacos

- Dinner: Stuffed Acorn Squash with Wild Rice

- Snack: Vegan Spinach Artichoke Dip

- Dessert: Chia Seed Chocolate Pudding

Week 4

Day 22

- Breakfast: Buckwheat Porridge with Cinnamon

- Lunch: Quinoa Stuffed Portobello Mushrooms

- Dinner: Vegan Pad Thai

- Snack: Coconut Yogurt with Fresh Berries

- Dessert: Blueberry Oat Bars

Day 23

- Breakfast: Almond Butter Overnight Oats

- Lunch: Thai Peanut Noodle Salad

- Dinner: Portobello Mushroom Burgers

- Snack: Trail Mix with Nuts and Seeds

- Dessert: Coconut Macaroons

Day 24

- Breakfast: Sweet Potato Hash with Kale

- Lunch: Vegan Minestrone Soup

- Dinner: Lentil Bolognese with Whole Wheat Pasta

- Snack: Veggie Sushi Rolls

- Dessert: Vegan Carrot Cake

Day 25

- Breakfast: Breakfast Quinoa with Coconut Milk

- Lunch: Falafel Wrap with Hummus

- Dinner: Moroccan Chickpea Stew

- Snack: Baked Sweet Potato Fries

- Dessert: Peanut Butter Chocolate Chip Blondies

Day 26

- Breakfast: Oatmeal with Berries and Almonds

- Lunch: Lentil and Vegetable Soup

- Dinner: Eggplant Parmesan

- Snack: Hummus and Crudites

- Dessert: Vegan Chocolate Avocado Mousse

Day 27

- Breakfast: Tofu Scramble with Spinach and Tomatoes
- Lunch: Chickpea Salad with Lemon Dressing
- Dinner: Cauliflower Steak with Chimichurri
- Snack: Edamame with Sea Salt
- Dessert: Berry Coconut Parfait

Day 28

- Breakfast: Chia Seed Pudding with Fresh Fruit
- Lunch: Stuffed Bell Peppers with Quinoa and Black Beans
- Dinner: Vegan Chili with Quinoa
- Snack: Guacamole with Whole Grain Tortilla Chips
- Dessert: Pumpkin Pie Energy Bites

Day 29

- Breakfast: Whole Grain Pancakes with Maple Syrup
- Lunch: Vegan Caesar Salad with Tofu
- Dinner: Ratatouille with Polenta
- Snack: Stuffed Dates with Almond Butter
- Dessert: Banana Nice Cream

Day 30

- Breakfast: Avocado Toast with Chickpeas
- Lunch: Spinach and Mushroom Quesadilla

- Dinner: Mushroom and Spinach Risotto
- Snack: Roasted Chickpeas with Paprika
- Dessert: Vegan Lemon Bars

Chapter 2: Breakfast Recipes

In the early hours of the day, a nourishing breakfast sets the tone for a healthy lifestyle. These 15 diverse breakfast recipes cater to both taste and health, ideal for those embracing a vegetarian or vegan diet.

Oatmeal with Berries and Almonds

Ingredients:

- 1/2 cup rolled oats
- 1 cup almond milk
- 1/2 cup mixed berries (strawberries, blueberries, raspberries)
- 2 tablespoons sliced almonds

Instructions:

1. Cook oats with almond milk until creamy.
2. Top with mixed berries and sliced almonds.
3. Serve warm.

Nutrition Information (per serving):

- Calories: 250
- Protein: 7g
- Carbohydrates: 40g

- Fat: 8g
- Fiber: 8g
- Sugar: 8g
- Portion size: 1 bowl

Tofu Scramble with Spinach and Tomatoes

Ingredients:

- 1/2 block tofu, crumbled
- 1 cup spinach, chopped
- 1 tomato, diced
- 1/2 teaspoon turmeric powder
- Salt and pepper to taste

Instructions:

1. Sauté tofu in a pan until slightly browned.
2. Add spinach, tomatoes, turmeric, salt, and pepper.
3. Cook until spinach wilts.
4. Serve hot.

Nutrition Information (per serving):

- Calories: 180
- Protein: 14g

- Carbohydrates: 10g

- Fat: 10g

- Fiber: 5g

- Sugar: 3g

- Portion size: 1 plate

Chia Seed Pudding with Fresh Fruit

Ingredients:

- 1/4 cup chia seeds

- 1 cup almond milk

- 1 tablespoon maple syrup (optional)

- Fresh mixed fruit (such as berries, mango, kiwi)

Instructions:

1. Mix chia seeds and almond milk in a bowl.

2. Let it sit for 15 minutes, stirring occasionally.

3. Sweeten with maple syrup if desired.

4. Top with fresh fruit before serving.

Nutrition Information (per serving):

- Calories: 220

- Protein: 6g

- Carbohydrates: 25g

- Fat: 10g
- Fiber: 12g
- Sugar: 10g
- Portion size: 1 bowl

Whole Grain Pancakes with Maple Syrup

Ingredients:

- 1 cup whole wheat flour
- 1 tablespoon baking powder
- 1 tablespoon maple syrup
- 1 cup almond milk

Instructions:

1. Mix flour and baking powder in a bowl.
2. Add maple syrup and almond milk, stir until smooth.
3. Heat a non-stick pan over medium heat.
4. Pour batter onto the pan and cook until bubbles form.
5. Flip and cook until golden brown.
6. Serve warm with additional maple syrup.

Nutrition Information (per serving):

- Calories: 180
- Protein: 6g

- Carbohydrates: 35g
- Fat: 2g
- Fiber: 4g
- Sugar: 6g
- Portion size: 2 pancakes

Avocado Toast with Chickpeas

Ingredients:

- 1 ripe avocado
- 1/2 cup canned chickpeas, rinsed and drained
- 2 slices whole grain bread
- Salt and pepper to taste

Instructions:

1. Mash avocado and spread evenly on toasted bread slices.
2. Top with chickpeas.
3. Season with salt and pepper.
4. Serve immediately.

Nutrition Information (per serving):

- Calories: 320
- Protein: 10g
- Carbohydrates: 40g

- Fat: 15g
- Fiber: 12g
- Sugar: 3g
- Portion size: 2 slices of toast

Vegan Breakfast Burrito

Ingredients:

- 1/2 cup black beans, cooked and drained
- 1/2 cup tofu, crumbled
- 1/2 cup bell peppers, diced
- 1/4 cup onion, diced
- 1/2 teaspoon cumin
- Salt and pepper to taste
- Whole grain tortillas

Instructions:

1. Sauté tofu, bell peppers, and onion in a pan until tender.
2. Add black beans, cumin, salt, and pepper, cook until heated through.
3. Warm tortillas and fill with the mixture.
4. Roll up burritos and serve.

Nutrition Information (per serving):

- Calories: 280
- Protein: 15g
- Carbohydrates: 40g
- Fat: 8g
- Fiber: 10g
- Sugar: 2g
- Portion size: 1 burrito

Quinoa Breakfast Bowl

Ingredients:

- 1 cup cooked quinoa
- 1/2 cup mixed berries
- 1 tablespoon almond butter
- 1 tablespoon honey or maple syrup (optional)
- Almond milk or yogurt (optional)

Instructions:

1. Place quinoa in a bowl.
2. Top with mixed berries, almond butter, and sweetener if desired.
3. Add almond milk or yogurt if desired.
4. Mix well and serve.

Nutrition Information (per serving):

- Calories: 300

- Protein: 10g

- Carbohydrates: 45g

- Fat: 8g

- Fiber: 6g

- Sugar: 12g

- Portion size: 1 bowl

Fruit and Nut Granola

Ingredients:

- 2 cups rolled oats

- 1/2 cup nuts (almonds, walnuts, etc.), chopped

- 1/4 cup seeds (pumpkin, sunflower, etc.)

- 1/4 cup dried fruit (raisins, cranberries, etc.)

- 1/4 cup maple syrup or honey

- 1/4 cup coconut oil, melted

- 1 teaspoon vanilla extract

- Pinch of salt

Instructions:

1. Preheat oven to 300°F (150°C) and line a baking sheet with parchment paper.

2. In a large bowl, combine oats, nuts, seeds, and dried fruit.

3. In a separate bowl, whisk together maple syrup (or honey), coconut oil, vanilla extract, and salt.

4. Pour wet ingredients over dry ingredients and mix until evenly coated.

5. Spread mixture onto the baking sheet in an even layer.

6. Bake for 30-35 minutes, stirring halfway through, until golden brown.

7. Allow granola to cool completely before breaking into clusters.

8. Store in an airtight container.

Nutrition Information (per serving, approximately 1/2 cup):

- Calories: 300
- Protein: 7g
- Carbohydrates: 30g
- Fat: 18g
- Fiber: 5g
- Sugar: 10g
- Portion size: 1/2 cup

Smoothie Bowl with Greens and Berries

Ingredients:

- 1 cup fresh spinach or kale
- 1 frozen banana
- 1/2 cup mixed berries (strawberries, blueberries, raspberries)
- 1/2 cup almond milk or coconut water
- Toppings: sliced fresh fruit, granola, chia seeds

Instructions:

1. Blend spinach or kale, frozen banana, mixed berries, and almond milk until smooth.
2. Pour into a bowl.
3. Top with sliced fresh fruit, granola, and chia seeds.
4. Serve immediately with a spoon.

Nutrition Information (per serving):

- Calories: 250
- Protein: 5g
- Carbohydrates: 55g
- Fat: 4g
- Fiber: 10g
- Sugar: 25g
- Portion size: 1 bowl

Vegan French Toast

Ingredients:

- 4 slices whole grain bread
- 1/2 cup almond milk
- 1 tablespoon ground flaxseed
- 1 teaspoon vanilla extract
- 1/2 teaspoon cinnamon
- Coconut oil for cooking
- Fresh fruit and maple syrup for serving

Instructions:

1. In a shallow bowl, whisk together almond milk, ground flaxseed, vanilla extract, and cinnamon.
2. Heat coconut oil in a non-stick skillet over medium heat.
3. Dip each slice of bread into the almond milk mixture, ensuring both sides are coated.
4. Place bread slices in the skillet and cook until golden brown on both sides.
5. Serve hot with fresh fruit and maple syrup.

Nutrition Information (per serving):

- Calories: 280
- Protein: 8g
- Carbohydrates: 40g

- Fat: 10g

- Fiber: 6g

- Sugar: 8g

- Portion size: 2 slices

Buckwheat Porridge with Cinnamon

Ingredients:

- 1/2 cup buckwheat groats

- 1 cup almond milk

- 1 tablespoon maple syrup or honey

- 1/2 teaspoon ground cinnamon

- Fresh berries or sliced banana for topping

Instructions:

1. Rinse buckwheat groats under cold water.

2. In a saucepan, bring almond milk to a boil.

3. Add buckwheat groats, reduce heat, and simmer for 15-20 minutes until tender.

4. Stir in maple syrup (or honey) and cinnamon.

5. Serve warm, topped with fresh berries or sliced banana.

Nutrition Information (per serving):

- Calories: 280

- Protein: 8g

- Carbohydrates: 50g

- Fat: 5g

- Fiber: 6g

- Sugar: 8g

- Portion size: 1 bowl

Vegan Banana Bread

Ingredients:

- 3 ripe bananas, mashed

- 1/4 cup almond milk

- 1/4 cup coconut oil, melted

- 1/2 cup maple syrup or agave nectar

- 1 teaspoon vanilla extract

- 2 cups whole wheat flour

- 1 teaspoon baking soda

- 1/2 teaspoon cinnamon

- Pinch of salt

- Optional: chopped nuts or chocolate chips

Instructions:

1. Preheat oven to 350°F (175°C) and grease a loaf pan.

2. In a large bowl, mix mashed bananas, almond milk, coconut oil, maple syrup (or agave nectar), and vanilla extract.

3. In another bowl, whisk together whole wheat flour, baking soda, cinnamon, and salt.

4. Combine wet and dry ingredients until just mixed. Fold in optional nuts or chocolate chips if using.

5. Pour batter into the loaf pan and spread evenly.

6. Bake for 50-60 minutes, or until a toothpick inserted into the center comes out clean.

7. Allow banana bread to cool in the pan for 10 minutes before transferring to a wire rack to cool completely.

Nutrition Information (per serving, based on 12 servings):

- Calories: 220
- Protein: 4g
- Carbohydrates: 35g
- Fat: 8g
- Fiber: 4g
- Sugar: 16g
- Portion size: 1 slice

Almond Butter Overnight Oats

Ingredients:

- 1/2 cup rolled oats
- 1 tablespoon almond butter
- 1/2 cup almond milk
- 1 tablespoon maple syrup or honey
- Sliced bananas or berries for topping

Instructions:

1. In a jar or bowl, combine rolled oats, almond butter, almond milk, and maple syrup (or honey).
2. Stir well to mix thoroughly.
3. Cover and refrigerate overnight or at least 4 hours.
4. Before serving, stir again and top with sliced bananas or berries.

Nutrition Information (per serving):

- Calories: 300
- Protein: 8g
- Carbohydrates: 40g
- Fat: 12g
- Fiber: 6g
- Sugar: 10g
- Portion size: 1 bowl

Sweet Potato Hash with Kale

Ingredients:

- 1 large sweet potato, peeled and diced
- 1 cup kale, chopped
- 1/2 onion, diced
- 1 garlic clove, minced
- 1/2 teaspoon paprika
- Salt and pepper to taste
- Olive oil for cooking

Instructions:

1. Heat olive oil in a skillet over medium heat.
2. Add diced sweet potato and cook for 5-7 minutes until slightly tender.
3. Add diced onion and minced garlic, cook until onion is translucent.
4. Stir in chopped kale, paprika, salt, and pepper.
5. Cook for another 5 minutes until kale is wilted and sweet potatoes are cooked through.
6. Serve hot.

Nutrition Information (per serving):

- Calories: 250
- Protein: 5g

- Carbohydrates: 40g
- Fat: 8g
- Fiber: 8g
- Sugar: 8g
- Portion size: 1 plate

Breakfast Quinoa with Coconut Milk

Ingredients:

- 1 cup quinoa
- 1 can (14 oz) coconut milk
- 1/2 cup water
- 1 tablespoon maple syrup or honey
- 1/2 teaspoon vanilla extract
- Fresh fruit for topping (such as mango, pineapple, or berries)
- Toasted coconut flakes (optional)

Instructions:

1. Rinse quinoa under cold water.
2. In a saucepan, combine quinoa, coconut milk, and water.
3. Bring to a boil, then reduce heat to low, cover, and simmer for 15-20 minutes until quinoa is cooked and liquid is absorbed.
4. Stir in maple syrup (or honey) and vanilla extract.

5. Serve warm, topped with fresh fruit and toasted coconut flakes if desired.

Nutrition Information (per serving):

- Calories: 350
- Protein: 8g
- Carbohydrates: 45g
- Fat: 15g
- Fiber: 4g
- Sugar: 8g
- Portion size: 1 bowl

Chapter 3: Lunch Recipes

These recipes are packed with wholesome ingredients that are not only satisfying but also beneficial for maintaining stable blood sugar levels. From hearty soups to vibrant salads and satisfying wraps, these lunches will keep you energized throughout the day. Each recipe includes essential nutrition information to help you make informed choices about your meals.

Lentil and Vegetable Soup

Ingredients:

- 1 cup green lentils, rinsed
- 2 carrots, diced
- 2 celery stalks, diced
- 1 onion, chopped
- 2 cloves garlic, minced
- 1 can (14 oz) diced tomatoes
- 4 cups vegetable broth
- 1 tsp dried thyme
- Salt and pepper to taste

Instructions:

1. In a large pot, sauté onion and garlic until fragrant.

2. Add carrots, celery, and lentils. Cook for 5 minutes.

3. Stir in diced tomatoes, vegetable broth, thyme, salt, and pepper.

4. Bring to a boil, then reduce heat and simmer for 30 minutes or until lentils are tender.

5. Serve hot.

Nutrition Information per serving:

- Calories: 250
- Protein: 15g
- Carbohydrates: 45g
- Fat: 1g
- Fiber: 15g
- Sugar: 8g
- Portion size: 1.5 cups

Chickpea Salad with Lemon Dressing

Ingredients:

- 1 can (15 oz) chickpeas, drained and rinsed
- 1 cucumber, diced
- 1 bell pepper, diced
- 1/4 cup red onion, finely chopped
- 1/4 cup fresh parsley, chopped

- Juice of 1 lemon

- 2 tbsp olive oil

- Salt and pepper to taste

Instructions:

1. In a large bowl, combine chickpeas, cucumber, bell pepper, red onion, and parsley.
2. In a small bowl, whisk together lemon juice, olive oil, salt, and pepper.
3. Pour dressing over salad and toss gently to combine.
4. Chill for at least 30 minutes before serving.

Nutrition Information per serving:

- Calories: 280

- Protein: 10g

- Carbohydrates: 35g

- Fat: 12g

- Fiber: 9g

- Sugar: 8g

- Portion size: 1 cup

Stuffed Bell Peppers with Quinoa and Black Beans

Ingredients:

- 4 bell peppers, any color
- 1 cup quinoa, cooked
- 1 can (15 oz) black beans, drained and rinsed
- 1 cup corn kernels
- 1/2 cup diced tomatoes
- 1/2 cup diced red onion
- 1 tsp cumin
- Salt and pepper to taste
- Fresh cilantro, for garnish

Instructions:

1. Preheat oven to 375°F (190°C). Cut tops off bell peppers and remove seeds.
2. In a large bowl, mix together quinoa, black beans, corn, tomatoes, red onion, cumin, salt, and pepper.
3. Stuff each bell pepper with quinoa mixture and place in a baking dish.
4. Cover with foil and bake for 30-35 minutes, until peppers are tender.
5. Garnish with fresh cilantro before serving.

Nutrition Information per serving:

- Calories: 320
- Protein: 12g
- Carbohydrates: 60g
- Fat: 3g
- Fiber: 12g
- Sugar: 8g
- Portion size: 1 stuffed pepper

Vegan Caesar Salad with Tofu

Ingredients:

- 1 block (14 oz) firm tofu, pressed and cubed
- 1 head romaine lettuce, chopped
- 1/2 cup vegan Caesar dressing
- 1/4 cup nutritional yeast
- 1 cup croutons (optional)
- Salt and pepper to taste

Instructions:

1. In a large bowl, toss cubed tofu with nutritional yeast, salt, and pepper.
2. Heat a non-stick skillet over medium heat and cook tofu until golden brown, about 5-7 minutes.

3. In a separate bowl, combine romaine lettuce and Caesar dressing. Toss to coat evenly.

4. Top salad with crispy tofu and croutons, if using.

5. Serve immediately.

Nutrition Information per serving:

- Calories: 280
- Protein: 18g
- Carbohydrates: 20g
- Fat: 15g
- Fiber: 6g
- Sugar: 4g
- Portion size: 2 cups salad

Spinach and Mushroom Quesadilla

Ingredients:

- 4 large whole wheat tortillas
- 2 cups spinach leaves
- 1 cup mushrooms, sliced
- 1/2 cup shredded vegan cheese
- 1/4 cup salsa
- Cooking spray or olive oil

Instructions:

1. Heat a non-stick skillet over medium heat.

2. Spray one side of a tortilla with cooking spray or brush with olive oil. Place it in the skillet, sprayed/oiled side down.

3. Layer spinach, mushrooms, and vegan cheese on half of the tortilla.

4. Fold the tortilla in half and press down gently with a spatula.

5. Cook for 2-3 minutes on each side, until tortilla is golden brown and crispy.

6. Repeat with remaining tortillas and filling ingredients.

7. Serve quesadillas hot with salsa on the side.

Nutrition Information per serving:

- Calories: 320
- Protein: 12g
- Carbohydrates: 40g
- Fat: 12g
- Fiber: 6g
- Sugar: 4g
- Portion size: 1 quesadilla

Mediterranean Couscous Salad

Ingredients:

- 1 cup couscous, cooked
- 1 cucumber, diced
- 1 bell pepper, diced
- 1/2 cup cherry tomatoes, halved
- 1/4 cup Kalamata olives, sliced
- 1/4 cup red onion, finely chopped
- 1/4 cup fresh parsley, chopped
- Juice of 1 lemon
- 2 tbsp olive oil
- Salt and pepper to taste

Instructions:

1. In a large bowl, combine cooked couscous, cucumber, bell pepper, cherry tomatoes, Kalamata olives, red onion, and parsley.
2. In a small bowl, whisk together lemon juice, olive oil, salt, and pepper.
3. Pour dressing over salad and toss gently to combine.
4. Chill for at least 30 minutes before serving.

Nutrition Information per serving:

- Calories: 280

- Protein: 8g

- Carbohydrates: 45g

- Fat: 8g

- Fiber: 5g

- Sugar: 3g

- Portion size: 1 cup

Sweet Potato and Black Bean Tacos

Ingredients:

- 4 small sweet potatoes, peeled and diced

- 1 can (15 oz) black beans, drained and rinsed

- 1 tbsp olive oil

- 1 tsp chili powder

- 1/2 tsp cumin

- Salt and pepper to taste

- 8 small corn or flour tortillas

- Toppings: shredded lettuce, diced tomatoes, avocado slices, salsa

Instructions:

1. Preheat oven to 400°F (200°C). Toss sweet potatoes with olive oil, chili powder, cumin, salt, and pepper.

2. Spread sweet potatoes on a baking sheet and roast for 20-25 minutes, until tender and slightly caramelized.

3. Heat black beans in a small saucepan over medium heat until warmed through.

4. Warm tortillas in a dry skillet or microwave.

5. Assemble tacos with roasted sweet potatoes, black beans, and desired toppings.

6. Serve immediately.

Nutrition Information per serving:

- Calories: 320
- Protein: 10g
- Carbohydrates: 60g
- Fat: 5g
- Fiber: 10g
- Sugar: 8g
- Portion size: 2 tacos

Vegan Buddha Bowl

Ingredients:

- 1 cup cooked quinoa or brown rice
- 1 cup roasted sweet potatoes
- 1 cup steamed broccoli florets

- 1 cup chickpeas, roasted with paprika
- 1/2 avocado, sliced
- 1/4 cup hummus
- Lemon tahini dressing (optional)

Instructions:

1. Arrange quinoa or brown rice, roasted sweet potatoes, steamed broccoli, chickpeas, and avocado in a bowl.
2. Drizzle with hummus and lemon tahini dressing, if desired.
3. Serve immediately.

Nutrition Information per serving:

- Calories: 450
- Protein: 15g
- Carbohydrates: 65g
- Fat: 18g
- Fiber: 15g
- Sugar: 5g
- Portion size: 1 bowl

Zucchini Noodles with Pesto

Ingredients:

- 4 medium zucchinis, spiralized into noodles

- 1/2 cup basil pesto (store-bought or homemade)
- Cherry tomatoes, halved, for garnish
- Pine nuts, toasted, for garnish
- Fresh basil leaves, for garnish

Instructions:

1. Heat a large skillet over medium heat. Add spiralized zucchini noodles and sauté for 2-3 minutes until just tender.
2. Toss the zucchini noodles with basil pesto until well coated.
3. Remove from heat and divide into serving bowls.
4. Garnish with cherry tomatoes, toasted pine nuts, and fresh basil leaves.
5. Serve immediately.

Nutrition Information per serving:

- Calories: 250
- Protein: 8g
- Carbohydrates: 15g
- Fat: 20g
- Fiber: 5g
- Sugar: 5g
- Portion size: 1.5 cups

Greek Salad with Tofu Feta

Ingredients:

- 1 block (14 oz) firm tofu, drained and cubed
- 1 cucumber, diced
- 1 bell pepper, diced
- 1/2 cup cherry tomatoes, halved
- 1/4 cup Kalamata olives, sliced
- 1/4 cup red onion, thinly sliced
- 1/4 cup fresh parsley, chopped
- Juice of 1 lemon
- 2 tbsp olive oil
- 1 tsp dried oregano
- Salt and pepper to taste

Instructions:

1. In a large bowl, combine tofu cubes, cucumber, bell pepper, cherry tomatoes, Kalamata olives, red onion, and parsley.
2. In a small bowl, whisk together lemon juice, olive oil, dried oregano, salt, and pepper.
3. Pour dressing over salad and toss gently to combine.
4. Chill for at least 30 minutes before serving.

Nutrition Information per serving:

- Calories: 280

- Protein: 15g
- Carbohydrates: 15g
- Fat: 18g
- Fiber: 5g
- Sugar: 5g
- Portion size: 1 cup

Quinoa Stuffed Portobello Mushrooms

Ingredients:

- 4 large Portobello mushrooms, stems removed
- 1 cup quinoa, cooked
- 1 cup baby spinach, chopped
- 1/2 cup sun-dried tomatoes, chopped
- 1/4 cup pine nuts, toasted
- 1/4 cup vegan Parmesan cheese (optional)
- Salt and pepper to taste

Instructions:

1. Preheat oven to 375°F (190°C). Place Portobello mushrooms on a baking sheet, gill side up.
2. In a bowl, mix together cooked quinoa, baby spinach, sun-dried tomatoes, pine nuts, vegan Parmesan (if using), salt, and pepper.

3. Spoon quinoa mixture into each mushroom cap, pressing gently to pack.

4. Bake for 20-25 minutes until mushrooms are tender and filling is heated through.

5. Serve hot.

Nutrition Information per serving:

- Calories: 320

- Protein: 12g

- Carbohydrates: 45g

- Fat: 10g

- Fiber: 8g

- Sugar: 5g

- Portion size: 1 stuffed mushroom

Thai Peanut Noodle Salad

Ingredients:

- 8 oz whole wheat spaghetti or rice noodles

- 1 cup shredded carrots

- 1 bell pepper, thinly sliced

- 1/2 cucumber, julienned

- 1/4 cup fresh cilantro, chopped

- 1/4 cup peanuts, chopped (optional for garnish)

For the Peanut Dressing:

- 1/4 cup peanut butter
- 2 tbsp soy sauce or tamari
- 2 tbsp rice vinegar
- 1 tbsp maple syrup or agave syrup
- 1 tbsp lime juice
- 1 clove garlic, minced
- 1 tsp grated ginger
- 1/4 cup water, as needed to thin the dressing

Instructions:

1. Cook noodles according to package instructions. Drain and rinse under cold water.
2. In a large bowl, combine cooked noodles, shredded carrots, bell pepper, cucumber, and cilantro.
3. In a separate bowl, whisk together all ingredients for the peanut dressing until smooth. Add water gradually to achieve desired consistency.
4. Pour dressing over the noodle salad and toss to coat evenly.
5. Garnish with chopped peanuts, if using, before serving.

Nutrition Information per serving:

- Calories: 380
- Protein: 12g

- Carbohydrates: 55g

- Fat: 15g

- Fiber: 8g

- Sugar: 8g

- Portion size: 2 cups

Vegan Minestrone Soup

Ingredients:

- 1 tbsp olive oil

- 1 onion, diced

- 2 cloves garlic, minced

- 2 carrots, diced

- 2 celery stalks, diced

- 1 zucchini, diced

- 1 can (15 oz) diced tomatoes

- 1 can (15 oz) kidney beans, drained and rinsed

- 4 cups vegetable broth

- 1 tsp dried oregano

- 1 tsp dried basil

- Salt and pepper to taste

- 1 cup whole wheat pasta, such as elbows or shells

- Fresh parsley, chopped, for garnish

Instructions:

1. In a large pot, heat olive oil over medium heat. Add onion and garlic, sauté until fragrant.
2. Add carrots, celery, and zucchini. Cook for 5 minutes until vegetables begin to soften.
3. Stir in diced tomatoes, kidney beans, vegetable broth, oregano, basil, salt, and pepper. Bring to a boil.
4. Reduce heat, cover, and simmer for 15-20 minutes until vegetables are tender.
5. Stir in pasta and cook according to package instructions until al dente.
6. Remove from heat and let soup stand for 5 minutes before serving.
7. Garnish with fresh parsley before serving.

Nutrition Information per serving:
- Calories: 320
- Protein: 12g
- Carbohydrates: 55g
- Fat: 6g
- Fiber: 12g
- Sugar: 8g
- Portion size: 1.5 cups

Falafel Wrap with Hummus

Ingredients:

- 4 whole wheat or gluten-free wraps
- 12 falafel balls, homemade or store-bought
- 1 cup shredded lettuce
- 1/2 cup diced tomatoes
- 1/2 cucumber, thinly sliced
- 1/4 cup sliced red onion
- 1/4 cup hummus
- Fresh parsley, chopped, for garnish

Instructions:

1. Warm falafel balls according to package instructions.
2. Heat wraps in a dry skillet until warm and flexible.
3. Spread hummus evenly over each wrap.
4. Divide shredded lettuce, diced tomatoes, cucumber slices, and red onion among the wraps.
5. Place falafel balls on top of the vegetables.
6. Garnish with fresh parsley.
7. Fold wraps tightly and serve immediately.

Nutrition Information per serving:

- Calories: 380
- Protein: 15g

- Carbohydrates: 55g

- Fat: 12g

- Fiber: 10g

- Sugar: 5g

- Portion size: 1 wrap

Vegan Sushi Rolls

Ingredients:

- 4 nori seaweed sheets

- 1 cup sushi rice, cooked and seasoned with rice vinegar

- 1/2 cucumber, julienned

- 1/2 avocado, sliced

- 1/2 carrot, julienned

- 1/2 red bell pepper, julienned

- Soy sauce, for serving

- Pickled ginger and wasabi, optional for serving

Instructions:

1. Place a nori sheet on a bamboo sushi mat or a clean kitchen towel.

2. Spread a thin layer of seasoned sushi rice evenly over the nori sheet, leaving a small border at the top edge.

3. Arrange cucumber, avocado, carrot, and bell pepper in a line across the center of the rice.

4. Using the sushi mat or towel, tightly roll the nori sheet over the filling, pressing gently to seal.

5. Moisten the top edge of the nori sheet with water to help seal the roll.

6. Repeat with remaining nori sheets and filling ingredients.

7. Slice each roll into 6-8 pieces using a sharp knife.

8. Serve sushi rolls with soy sauce, pickled ginger, and wasabi if desired.

Nutrition Information per serving (4 pieces):

- Calories: 280
- Protein: 6g
- Carbohydrates: 55g
- Fat: 4g
- Fiber: 5g
- Sugar: 3g
- Portion size: 4 pieces

Chapter 4: Dinner Recipes

In this chapter, you'll discover a variety of hearty and nutritious dinner options suitable for vegetarians and vegans managing prediabetes. Each recipe is crafted to be flavorful and satisfying while supporting your dietary needs. From comforting pasta dishes to vibrant curries and savory stuffed vegetables, these recipes are designed to inspire your meal planning and promote balanced eating habits.

Eggplant Parmesan

Ingredients:

- 2 medium eggplants, sliced
- 1 cup breadcrumbs (preferably whole grain)
- 1 cup marinara sauce
- 1 cup shredded vegan mozzarella cheese
- 1/4 cup grated vegan Parmesan cheese
- Fresh basil leaves for garnish
- Salt and pepper to taste

Instructions:

1. Preheat oven to 400°F (200°C).

2. Dip eggplant slices in breadcrumbs, ensuring they are evenly coated.

3. Place coated eggplant slices on a baking sheet lined with parchment paper. Bake for 20-25 minutes or until golden brown.

4. In a baking dish, spread a thin layer of marinara sauce. Arrange half of the baked eggplant slices on top.

5. Sprinkle with half of the mozzarella and Parmesan cheeses. Repeat layers with remaining ingredients.

6. Bake for an additional 20 minutes until cheese is melted and bubbly.

7. Garnish with fresh basil leaves before serving.

Nutrition Information (per serving):

- Calories: 320
- Protein: 12g
- Carbohydrates: 45g
- Fat: 10g
- Fiber: 10g
- Sugar: 12g
- Portion size: 1/6 of recipe

Cauliflower Steak with Chimichurri

Ingredients:

- 1 large cauliflower head, sliced into steaks
- 1/4 cup olive oil
- Salt and pepper to taste

Chimichurri sauce:

- 1 cup fresh parsley, chopped
- 1/4 cup fresh cilantro, chopped
- 2 cloves garlic, minced
- 2 tablespoons red wine vinegar
- 1/4 cup olive oil
- Salt and pepper to taste

Instructions:

1. Preheat grill or grill pan over medium-high heat.
2. Brush cauliflower steaks with olive oil and season with salt and pepper.
3. Grill cauliflower steaks for 5-7 minutes per side, or until tender and grill marks appear.
4. In a small bowl, combine parsley, cilantro, garlic, red wine vinegar, and olive oil to make chimichurri sauce. Season with salt and pepper.

5. Serve grilled cauliflower steaks drizzled with chimichurri
   sauce.

Nutrition Information (per serving):

- Calories: 250
- Protein: 5g
- Carbohydrates: 15g
- Fat: 20g
- Fiber: 6g
- Sugar: 4g
- Portion size: 1/4 of recipe

Vegan Chili with Quinoa

Ingredients:

- 1 tablespoon olive oil
- 1 onion, diced
- 3 cloves garlic, minced
- 1 red bell pepper, diced
- 1 green bell pepper, diced
- 1 cup quinoa, rinsed
- 1 can (15 oz) black beans, drained and rinsed
- 1 can (15 oz) kidney beans, drained and rinsed
- 1 can (28 oz) crushed tomatoes

- 2 cups vegetable broth
- 2 tablespoons chili powder
- 1 teaspoon cumin
- Salt and pepper to taste
- Fresh cilantro for garnish

Instructions:

1. Heat olive oil in a large pot over medium heat. Add onion and garlic, sauté until softened.
2. Add bell peppers and cook for 3-4 minutes until slightly tender.
3. Stir in quinoa, black beans, kidney beans, crushed tomatoes, vegetable broth, chili powder, cumin, salt, and pepper.
4. Bring to a boil, then reduce heat to low. Cover and simmer for 20-25 minutes, or until quinoa is cooked and chili has thickened.
5. Adjust seasoning if needed. Serve hot, garnished with fresh cilantro.

Nutrition Information (per serving):

- Calories: 350
- Protein: 15g
- Carbohydrates: 60g
- Fat: 5g

- Fiber: 15g
- Sugar: 10g
- Portion size: 1/6 of recipe

Ratatouille with Polenta

Ingredients:

- 1 eggplant, diced
- 1 zucchini, diced
- 1 yellow squash, diced
- 1 red bell pepper, diced
- 1 onion, diced
- 2 cloves garlic, minced
- 1 can (15 oz) diced tomatoes
- 1 tablespoon tomato paste
- 1 teaspoon dried thyme
- Salt and pepper to taste
- 1 tube (18 oz) pre-cooked polenta, sliced
- Fresh basil for garnish

Instructions:

1. Heat olive oil in a large skillet over medium heat. Add onion and garlic, sauté until translucent.

2. Add diced eggplant, zucchini, yellow squash, and bell pepper. Cook for 8-10 minutes until vegetables are tender.

3. Stir in diced tomatoes, tomato paste, dried thyme, salt, and pepper. Simmer for 10-15 minutes, stirring occasionally.

4. Meanwhile, heat a non-stick pan over medium heat. Fry polenta slices for 3-4 minutes per side until golden brown and crispy.

5. Serve ratatouille over crispy polenta slices, garnished with fresh basil.

Nutrition Information (per serving):

- Calories: 280
- Protein: 7g
- Carbohydrates: 45g
- Fat: 8g
- Fiber: 10g
- Sugar: 12g
- Portion size: 1/4 of recipe

Mushroom and Spinach Risotto

Ingredients:

- 1 tablespoon olive oil
- 1 onion, finely chopped

- 2 cloves garlic, minced

- 1 cup Arborio rice

- 1/2 cup dry white wine (optional)

- 4 cups vegetable broth, heated

- 8 oz cremini mushrooms, sliced

- 2 cups baby spinach leaves

- 1/4 cup nutritional yeast (optional for cheesy flavor)

- Salt and pepper to taste

- Fresh parsley for garnish

Instructions:

1. Heat olive oil in a large skillet over medium heat. Add onion and garlic, sauté until softened.

2. Stir in Arborio rice and cook for 2-3 minutes until translucent.

3. If using, pour in white wine and stir until absorbed.

4. Gradually add hot vegetable broth, one ladleful at a time, stirring frequently and allowing the liquid to absorb before adding more.

5. When rice is almost tender and creamy, stir in sliced mushrooms and continue cooking for 5-7 minutes.

6. Fold in baby spinach leaves and nutritional yeast (if using). Season with salt and pepper.

7. Remove from heat, cover, and let rest for 5 minutes before serving. Garnish with fresh parsley.

Nutrition Information (per serving):

- Calories: 320
- Protein: 8g
- Carbohydrates: 55g
- Fat: 6g
- Fiber: 4g
- Sugar: 3g
- Portion size: 1/4 of recipe

Butternut Squash Curry

Ingredients:

- 1 tablespoon coconut oil
- 1 onion, diced
- 3 cloves garlic, minced
- 1 tablespoon fresh ginger, minced
- 1 butternut squash, peeled, seeded, and cubed
- 1 can (15 oz) chickpeas, drained and rinsed
- 1 can (15 oz) coconut milk
- 1 cup vegetable broth
- 2 tablespoons red curry paste

- 1 tablespoon soy sauce or tamari
- 1 tablespoon maple syrup or coconut sugar
- Salt and pepper to taste
- Fresh cilantro for garnish

Instructions:

1. Heat coconut oil in a large pot over medium heat. Add onion, garlic, and ginger. Sauté until onion is translucent.
2. Add cubed butternut squash and chickpeas, stir to coat with oil and spices.
3. Pour in coconut milk and vegetable broth. Stir in red curry paste, soy sauce, and maple syrup.
4. Bring to a boil, then reduce heat and simmer uncovered for 20-25 minutes, or until butternut squash is tender.
5. Season with salt and pepper to taste. Serve hot, garnished with fresh cilantro.

Nutrition Information (per serving):

- Calories: 380
- Protein: 10g
- Carbohydrates: 45g
- Fat: 20g
- Fiber: 10g
- Sugar: 10g

- Portion size: 1/4 of recipe

Stuffed Acorn Squash with Wild Rice

Ingredients:

- 2 acorn squash, halved and seeded
- 1 tablespoon olive oil
- 1 onion, diced
- 2 cloves garlic, minced
- 1 cup wild rice, cooked
- 1/2 cup dried cranberries
- 1/2 cup pecans, chopped
- 1/4 cup fresh parsley, chopped
- Salt and pepper to taste

Instructions:

1. Preheat oven to 400°F (200°C).
2. Brush acorn squash halves with olive oil and place cut-side down on a baking sheet. Bake for 30 minutes, or until tender.
3. Meanwhile, heat olive oil in a skillet over medium heat. Add onion and garlic, sauté until softened.
4. Stir in cooked wild rice, dried cranberries, chopped pecans, and fresh parsley. Season with salt and pepper.
5. Fill each baked acorn squash half with the rice mixture.

6. Return stuffed squash to the oven and bake for an additional 10-15 minutes until heated through.

7. Serve hot as a main dish or side.

Nutrition Information (per serving):

- Calories: 320
- Protein: 6g
- Carbohydrates: 45g
- Fat: 15g
- Fiber: 8g
- Sugar: 10g
- Portion size: 1/2 of squash (1/4 of recipe)

Vegan Shepherd's Pie

Ingredients:

- 4 large potatoes, peeled and cubed
- 1/4 cup unsweetened almond milk or other non-dairy milk
- 2 tablespoons vegan butter
- Salt and pepper to taste
- 1 tablespoon olive oil
- 1 onion, diced
- 2 cloves garlic, minced
- 1 carrot, diced

- 1 celery stalk, diced
- 1 cup mushrooms, chopped
- 1 can (15 oz) lentils, drained and rinsed
- 1 cup frozen peas
- 1 cup vegetable broth
- 2 tablespoons tomato paste
- 1 teaspoon thyme
- 1 teaspoon rosemary
- Salt and pepper to taste

Instructions:

1. Preheat oven to 400°F (200°C).
2. Place potatoes in a large pot and cover with water. Bring to a boil, then reduce heat and simmer for 15-20 minutes, or until potatoes are tender.
3. Drain potatoes and return to pot. Mash with almond milk, vegan butter, salt, and pepper until smooth and creamy. Set aside.
4. Meanwhile, heat olive oil in a large skillet over medium heat. Add onion and garlic, sauté until softened.
5. Add diced carrot, celery, and mushrooms. Cook for 5-7 minutes until vegetables are tender.

6. Stir in lentils, frozen peas, vegetable broth, tomato paste, thyme, rosemary, salt, and pepper. Simmer for 10 minutes, stirring occasionally.

7. Transfer lentil mixture to a baking dish. Spread mashed potatoes evenly over the top.

8. Bake for 25-30 minutes, or until the top is golden brown.

9. Let cool for 5 minutes before serving.

Nutrition Information (per serving):

- Calories: 380
- Protein: 12g
- Carbohydrates: 65g
- Fat: 8g
- Fiber: 15g
- Sugar: 8g
- Portion size: 1/6 of recipe

Lemon Garlic Pasta with Asparagus

Ingredients:

- 8 oz whole wheat pasta
- 1 tablespoon olive oil
- 3 cloves garlic, minced
- 1 bunch asparagus, trimmed and cut into 2-inch pieces

- Zest and juice of 1 lemon
- 1/4 cup chopped fresh parsley
- Salt and pepper to taste
- Red pepper flakes (optional)

Instructions:

1. Cook pasta according to package instructions until al dente. Drain and set aside.
2. Heat olive oil in a large skillet over medium heat. Add minced garlic and cook for 1 minute until fragrant.
3. Add asparagus pieces to the skillet and sauté for 5-7 minutes until tender-crisp.
4. Toss cooked pasta in the skillet with lemon zest, lemon juice, chopped parsley, salt, and pepper.
5. If desired, sprinkle with red pepper flakes for added spice.
6. Serve immediately, garnished with additional parsley if desired.

Nutrition Information (per serving):

- Calories: 320
- Protein: 12g
- Carbohydrates: 60g
- Fat: 6g
- Fiber: 8g

- Sugar: 4g
- Portion size: 1/4 of recipe

Black Bean and Sweet Potato Enchiladas

Ingredients:

- 1 tablespoon olive oil
- 1 onion, diced
- 2 cloves garlic, minced
- 2 sweet potatoes, peeled and diced
- 1 can (15 oz) black beans, drained and rinsed
- 1 teaspoon ground cumin
- 1 teaspoon chili powder
- Salt and pepper to taste
- 8 whole wheat tortillas
- 1 can (15 oz) enchilada sauce
- 1 cup shredded vegan cheese
- Fresh cilantro for garnish

Instructions:

1. Preheat oven to 375°F (190°C).
2. Heat olive oil in a large skillet over medium heat. Add onion and garlic, sauté until softened.

3. Add diced sweet potatoes to the skillet and cook for 8-10 minutes until tender.

4. Stir in black beans, ground cumin, chili powder, salt, and pepper. Cook for another 2-3 minutes until heated through.

5. Spoon a portion of the sweet potato and black bean mixture onto each tortilla. Roll up and place seam-side down in a baking dish.

6. Pour enchilada sauce evenly over the rolled tortillas. Sprinkle with shredded vegan cheese.

7. Bake for 20-25 minutes until cheese is melted and bubbly.

8. Garnish with fresh cilantro before serving.

Nutrition Information (per serving):

- Calories: 380
- Protein: 15g
- Carbohydrates: 55g
- Fat: 10g
- Fiber: 10g
- Sugar: 8g
- Portion size: 2 enchiladas (1/4 of recipe)

Vegan Pad Thai

Ingredients:

- 8 oz rice noodles
- 1 tablespoon sesame oil
- 1 onion, thinly sliced
- 2 cloves garlic, minced
- 1 bell pepper, thinly sliced
- 1 cup shredded cabbage
- 1 cup shredded carrots
- 1/2 cup tofu, cubed
- 1/4 cup chopped peanuts
- 2 tablespoons soy sauce or tamari
- 1 tablespoon maple syrup or coconut sugar
- Juice of 1 lime
- Fresh cilantro for garnish
- Lime wedges for serving

Instructions:

1. Cook rice noodles according to package instructions until al dente. Drain and set aside.
2. Heat sesame oil in a large skillet or wok over medium-high heat. Add onion and garlic, sauté until softened.

3. Add bell pepper, shredded cabbage, shredded carrots, and tofu cubes. Stir-fry for 5-7 minutes until vegetables are tender-crisp.

4. In a small bowl, whisk together soy sauce, maple syrup (or coconut sugar), and lime juice.

5. Add cooked rice noodles and sauce to the skillet. Toss everything together until well combined and heated through.

6. Remove from heat and sprinkle with chopped peanuts and fresh cilantro.

7. Serve hot with lime wedges on the side.

Nutrition Information (per serving):

- Calories: 400
- Protein: 12g
- Carbohydrates: 65g
- Fat: 10g
- Fiber: 6g
- Sugar: 10g
- Portion size: 1/4 of recipe

Portobello Mushroom Burgers

Ingredients:

- 4 large portobello mushroom caps

- 2 tablespoons balsamic vinegar

- 2 tablespoons soy sauce or tamari

- 2 tablespoons olive oil

- 1 teaspoon dried thyme

- 1 teaspoon smoked paprika

- Salt and pepper to taste

- 4 whole wheat burger buns

- Lettuce, tomato slices, avocado slices for serving

Instructions:

1. Clean portobello mushroom caps and remove stems.

2. In a shallow dish, whisk together balsamic vinegar, soy sauce, olive oil, dried thyme, smoked paprika, salt, and pepper.

3. Place mushroom caps in the marinade, turning to coat. Let marinate for at least 30 minutes, flipping halfway through.

4. Preheat grill or grill pan over medium-high heat. Grill mushroom caps for 4-5 minutes per side, or until tender and grill marks appear.

5. Toast burger buns on the grill for 1-2 minutes until lightly browned.

6. Assemble burgers with grilled portobello mushroom caps, lettuce, tomato slices, and avocado slices.

7. Serve immediately.

Nutrition Information (per serving, without bun):

- Calories: 150
- Protein: 8g
- Carbohydrates: 10g
- Fat: 10g
- Fiber: 3g
- Sugar: 5g
- Portion size: 1 mushroom cap

Lentil Bolognese with Whole Wheat Pasta

Ingredients:

- 8 oz whole wheat pasta
- 1 tablespoon olive oil
- 1 onion, diced
- 2 carrots, diced
- 2 celery stalks, diced
- 2 cloves garlic, minced
- 1 cup dried green lentils, rinsed
- 1 can (15 oz) crushed tomatoes
- 1 cup vegetable broth
- 1 teaspoon dried oregano
- 1 teaspoon dried basil

- Salt and pepper to taste
- Fresh parsley for garnish

Instructions:

1. Cook pasta according to package instructions until al dente. Drain and set aside.
2. Heat olive oil in a large skillet over medium heat. Add onion, carrots, and celery. Sauté until vegetables are softened, about 5-7 minutes.
3. Add minced garlic and cook for 1 minute until fragrant.
4. Stir in dried lentils, crushed tomatoes, vegetable broth, dried oregano, dried basil, salt, and pepper.
5. Bring to a boil, then reduce heat to low. Cover and simmer for 25-30 minutes, or until lentils are tender and sauce has thickened.
6. Adjust seasoning if needed. Serve lentil Bolognese over cooked whole wheat pasta, garnished with fresh parsley.

Nutrition Information (per serving):

- Calories: 350
- Protein: 15g
- Carbohydrates: 60g
- Fat: 5g
- Fiber: 12g

- Sugar: 8g
- Portion size: 1/4 of recipe

Moroccan Chickpea Stew

Ingredients:

- 1 tablespoon olive oil
- 1 onion, diced
- 3 cloves garlic, minced
- 1 tablespoon fresh ginger, minced
- 1 teaspoon ground cumin
- 1 teaspoon ground coriander
- 1/2 teaspoon ground cinnamon
- 1/4 teaspoon ground turmeric
- 1/4 teaspoon cayenne pepper (optional)
- 1 can (15 oz) chickpeas, drained and rinsed
- 1 can (15 oz) diced tomatoes
- 2 cups vegetable broth
- 1 sweet potato, peeled and diced
- 1 cup chopped kale or spinach
- Salt and pepper to taste
- Fresh cilantro for garnish

Instructions:

1. Heat olive oil in a large pot over medium heat. Add onion and sauté until softened.

2. Stir in garlic, ginger, ground cumin, ground coriander, ground cinnamon, ground turmeric, and cayenne pepper (if using). Cook for 1 minute until fragrant.

3. Add chickpeas, diced tomatoes (with juices), vegetable broth, and diced sweet potato. Bring to a boil.

4. Reduce heat to low, cover, and simmer for 20-25 minutes, or until sweet potato is tender.

5. Stir in chopped kale or spinach and cook for an additional 5 minutes until greens are wilted.

6. Season with salt and pepper to taste. Serve hot, garnished with fresh cilantro.

Nutrition Information (per serving):

- Calories: 300
- Protein: 12g
- Carbohydrates: 50g
- Fat: 7g
- Fiber: 12g
- Sugar: 10g
- Portion size: 1/4 of recipe

Spinach and Artichoke Stuffed Shells

Ingredients:

- 12 oz jumbo pasta shells
- 1 tablespoon olive oil
- 1 onion, diced
- 3 cloves garlic, minced
- 8 oz frozen spinach, thawed and squeezed dry
- 1 can (14 oz) artichoke hearts, drained and chopped
- 1 cup vegan ricotta cheese
- 1/2 cup nutritional yeast (optional for cheesy flavor)
- 1 teaspoon dried basil
- 1 teaspoon dried oregano
- Salt and pepper to taste
- 2 cups marinara sauce
- Fresh basil for garnish

Instructions:

1. Cook pasta shells according to package instructions until al dente. Drain and set aside.
2. Preheat oven to 375°F (190°C).
3. Heat olive oil in a large skillet over medium heat. Add onion and garlic, sauté until softened.
4. Stir in thawed spinach and chopped artichoke hearts. Cook for 3-4 minutes until heated through.

5. In a large bowl, combine spinach and artichoke mixture with vegan ricotta cheese, nutritional yeast (if using), dried basil, dried oregano, salt, and pepper.

6. Stuff cooked pasta shells with the spinach and artichoke filling.

7. Spread 1 cup of marinara sauce evenly on the bottom of a baking dish.

8. Arrange stuffed shells in the baking dish. Top with remaining marinara sauce.

9. Cover with foil and bake for 20-25 minutes until heated through.

10. Garnish with fresh basil before serving.

Nutrition Information (per serving):

- Calories: 380
- Protein: 15g
- Carbohydrates: 60g
- Fat: 10g
- Fiber: 8g
- Sugar: 10g
- Portion size: 3 shells

Chapter 5: Snacks and Appetizers

These recipes are not only tasty but also nutritious, making them ideal choices for those managing prediabetes on a vegetarian or vegan diet. Whether you're looking for a quick bite between meals or hosting a gathering, these snacks and appetizers will satisfy your cravings without compromising your health goals.

Hummus and Crudites

Ingredients:

- 1 cup hummus
- Assorted raw vegetables such as carrots, celery, bell peppers, and cucumber

Instructions:

1. Wash and prepare the vegetables by cutting them into sticks or bite-sized pieces.
2. Serve the hummus alongside the crudites for dipping.

Nutrition Information (per serving):

- Calories: 150
- Protein: 5g
- Carbohydrates: 15g

- Fat: 8g
- Fiber: 6g
- Sugar: 3g
- Portion size: 1/2 cup hummus with 1 cup vegetables

Edamame with Sea Salt

Ingredients:

- 2 cups edamame (frozen, thawed)
- Sea salt to taste

Instructions:

1. Steam or boil the edamame according to package instructions.
2. Drain and sprinkle with sea salt before serving.

Nutrition Information (per serving):

- Calories: 120
- Protein: 12g
- Carbohydrates: 9g
- Fat: 4g
- Fiber: 5g
- Sugar: 3g
- Portion size: 1 cup

Guacamole with Whole Grain Tortilla Chips

Ingredients:

- 2 ripe avocados
- 1 tomato, diced
- 1/4 cup onion, finely chopped
- 1/4 cup fresh cilantro, chopped
- Juice of 1 lime
- Salt and pepper to taste
- Whole grain tortilla chips for serving

Instructions:

1. In a bowl, mash the avocados with a fork until smooth.
2. Stir in the diced tomato, onion, cilantro, lime juice, salt, and pepper.
3. Serve with whole grain tortilla chips.

Nutrition Information (per serving):

- Calories: 180
- Protein: 4g
- Carbohydrates: 15g
- Fat: 12g
- Fiber: 7g
- Sugar: 2g

- Portion size: 1/2 cup guacamole with 10 tortilla chips

Stuffed Dates with Almond Butter

Ingredients:

- 15 Medjool dates, pitted
- Almond butter for filling

Instructions:

1. Gently open each date and remove the pit.
2. Fill each date with almond butter.
3. Serve immediately or refrigerate until ready to eat.

Nutrition Information (per serving, 2 dates):

- Calories: 160
- Protein: 2g
- Carbohydrates: 30g
- Fat: 6g
- Fiber: 4g
- Sugar: 26g
- Portion size: 2 dates

Roasted Chickpeas with Paprika

Ingredients:

- 2 cups cooked chickpeas
- 1 tablespoon olive oil
- 1 teaspoon paprika
- Salt to taste

Instructions:

1. Preheat oven to 400°F (200°C).
2. Pat dry chickpeas with a paper towel to remove excess moisture.
3. Toss chickpeas with olive oil, paprika, and salt.
4. Spread on a baking sheet and roast for 25-30 minutes until crispy.
5. Let cool before serving.

Nutrition Information (per serving, 1/2 cup):

- Calories: 180
- Protein: 8g
- Carbohydrates: 27g
- Fat: 5g
- Fiber: 8g
- Sugar: 5g
- Portion size: 1/2 cup

Caprese Skewers with Balsamic Glaze

Ingredients:

- Cherry tomatoes
- Fresh mozzarella balls (bocconcini)
- Fresh basil leaves
- Balsamic glaze

Instructions:

1. Thread one cherry tomato, one mozzarella ball, and one basil leaf onto each skewer.
2. Drizzle with balsamic glaze just before serving.

Nutrition Information (per serving, 2 skewers):

- Calories: 120
- Protein: 8g
- Carbohydrates: 5g
- Fat: 8g
- Fiber: 1g
- Sugar: 3g
- Portion size: 2 skewers

Vegan Spinach Artichoke Dip

Ingredients:

- 1 cup raw cashews, soaked and drained
- 1 cup unsweetened almond milk
- 1 tablespoon nutritional yeast
- 1 clove garlic, minced
- 1 tablespoon lemon juice
- 1/2 teaspoon salt
- 1 cup frozen spinach, thawed and drained
- 1 cup canned artichoke hearts, chopped

Instructions:

1. In a blender, combine cashews, almond milk, nutritional yeast, garlic, lemon juice, and salt. Blend until smooth.
2. Transfer mixture to a saucepan and heat over medium-low heat.
3. Stir in spinach and artichoke hearts, cooking until heated through.
4. Serve warm with whole grain crackers or crudites.

Nutrition Information (per serving, 1/4 cup dip):

- Calories: 150
- Protein: 6g
- Carbohydrates: 10g

- Fat: 10g

- Fiber: 3g

- Sugar: 2g

- Portion size: 1/4 cup dip

Sliced Apple with Nut Butter

Ingredients:

- 1 large apple, sliced

- Nut butter of your choice (almond, peanut, cashew, etc.)

Instructions:

1. Slice the apple into wedges or rounds.

2. Spread each slice with nut butter.

3. Arrange on a plate and serve.

Nutrition Information (per serving):

- Calories: 150

- Protein: 3g

- Carbohydrates: 20g

- Fat: 8g

- Fiber: 5g

- Sugar: 14g

- Portion size: 1 large apple with 2 tablespoons nut butter

Vegan Cheese and Crackers

Ingredients:

- Vegan cheese slices or wedges
- Whole grain crackers

Instructions:

1. Arrange vegan cheese and whole grain crackers on a serving platter.

Nutrition Information (per serving):

- Calories: 200
- Protein: 6g
- Carbohydrates: 25g
- Fat: 9g
- Fiber: 4g
- Sugar: 2g
- Portion size: 2 ounces cheese with 5 crackers

Quinoa and Black Bean Stuffed Mini Peppers

Ingredients:

- 15 mini bell peppers
- 1 cup cooked quinoa

- 1 cup black beans, drained and rinsed
- 1/2 cup salsa
- 1/2 teaspoon cumin
- Salt and pepper to taste

Instructions:

1. Preheat oven to 375°F (190°C).
2. Cut tops off mini peppers and remove seeds.
3. In a bowl, combine quinoa, black beans, salsa, cumin, salt, and pepper.
4. Stuff each mini pepper with quinoa mixture.
5. Place stuffed peppers on a baking sheet and bake for 15-20 minutes until peppers are tender.

Nutrition Information (per serving, 3 peppers):

- Calories: 180
- Protein: 7g
- Carbohydrates: 30g
- Fat: 3g
- Fiber: 7g
- Sugar: 5g
- Portion size: 3 stuffed peppers

Coconut Yogurt with Fresh Berries

Ingredients:

- 1 cup unsweetened coconut yogurt
- Assorted fresh berries (strawberries, blueberries, raspberries)

Instructions:

1. Spoon coconut yogurt into a bowl.
2. Top with fresh berries.

Nutrition Information (per serving):

- Calories: 120
- Protein: 2g
- Carbohydrates: 15g
- Fat: 5g
- Fiber: 3g
- Sugar: 10g
- Portion size: 1 cup yogurt with 1/2 cup berries

Trail Mix with Nuts and Seeds

Ingredients:

- 1 cup mixed nuts (almonds, cashews, walnuts)
- 1/2 cup mixed seeds (pumpkin seeds, sunflower seeds)

- 1/2 cup dried fruit (raisins, cranberries)

Instructions:

1. Combine nuts, seeds, and dried fruit in a bowl.
2. Mix well and portion into small snack bags or containers.

Nutrition Information (per serving, 1/4 cup):

- Calories: 200
- Protein: 8g
- Carbohydrates: 15g
- Fat: 12g
- Fiber: 4g
- Sugar: 8g
- Portion size: 1/4 cup

Veggie Sushi Rolls

Ingredients:

- Nori seaweed sheets
- Cooked sushi rice
- Assorted vegetables (cucumber, avocado, carrot, bell pepper)
- Soy sauce and wasabi for serving

Instructions:

1. Place a nori sheet on a bamboo sushi mat.
2. Spread a thin layer of sushi rice over the nori, leaving a border at the top.
3. Arrange vegetables in a line across the rice.
4. Roll the sushi tightly using the bamboo mat.
5. Slice into bite-sized pieces and serve with soy sauce and wasabi.

Nutrition Information (per serving, 6 pieces):

- Calories: 180
- Protein: 5g
- Carbohydrates: 35g
- Fat: 2g
- Fiber: 5g
- Sugar: 2g
- Portion size: 6 pieces

Baked Sweet Potato Fries

Ingredients:

- 2 large sweet potatoes, peeled and cut into fries
- 1 tablespoon olive oil
- 1/2 teaspoon paprika

- Salt and pepper to taste

Instructions:

1. Preheat oven to 425°F (220°C).
2. Toss sweet potato fries with olive oil, paprika, salt, and pepper in a bowl.
3. Spread fries in a single layer on a baking sheet.
4. Bake for 25-30 minutes, flipping halfway through, until fries are crispy.

Nutrition Information (per serving, 1 cup):

- Calories: 150
- Protein: 2g
- Carbohydrates: 30g
- Fat: 3g
- Fiber: 5g
- Sugar: 6g
- Portion size: 1 cup

Cucumber Avocado Rolls

Ingredients:

- 2 large cucumbers
- 1 avocado, sliced

- 1/4 cup shredded carrots
- 1/4 cup alfalfa sprouts
- 1 tablespoon sesame seeds
- Soy sauce or tamari for dipping

Instructions:

1. Using a vegetable peeler, slice cucumbers lengthwise into thin strips.
2. Lay cucumber strips flat and place avocado slices, shredded carrots, and alfalfa sprouts on one end.
3. Roll up tightly and secure with a toothpick if needed.
4. Sprinkle with sesame seeds and serve with soy sauce or tamari for dipping.

Nutrition Information (per serving, 4 rolls):

- Calories: 160
- Protein: 3g
- Carbohydrates: 15g
- Fat: 10g
- Fiber: 7g
- Sugar: 4g
- Portion size: 4 rolls

Chapter 6: Desserts

Indulge guilt-free with these delicious vegan desserts designed to satisfy your sweet tooth while supporting a healthy lifestyle. Each recipe is crafted with wholesome ingredients and simple instructions to ensure delightful results every time.

Vegan Chocolate Avocado Mousse

Ingredients:

- 2 ripe avocados
- 1/4 cup cocoa powder
- 1/4 cup maple syrup
- 1 tsp vanilla extract
- Pinch of salt

Instructions:

1. Blend all ingredients in a food processor until smooth.
2. Chill in the refrigerator for 30 minutes before serving.

Nutrition Information:

- Calories: 180
- Protein: 3g
- Carbohydrates: 20g

- Fat: 12g
- Fiber: 7g
- Sugar: 10g
- Portion size: 1/2 cup

Berry Coconut Parfait

Ingredients:

- 1 cup coconut yogurt
- 1 cup mixed berries (strawberries, blueberries, raspberries)
- 1/4 cup granola
- Drizzle of agave or maple syrup (optional)

Instructions:

1. Layer coconut yogurt, berries, and granola in a glass or bowl.
2. Repeat layers and top with a drizzle of syrup if desired.

Nutrition Information:

- Calories: 220
- Protein: 5g
- Carbohydrates: 35g
- Fat: 7g
- Fiber: 6g
- Sugar: 18g

- Portion size: 1 serving

Pumpkin Pie Energy Bites

Ingredients:

- 1 cup rolled oats
- 1/2 cup pumpkin puree
- 1/4 cup almond butter
- 2 tbsp maple syrup
- 1 tsp pumpkin pie spice

Instructions:

1. Mix all ingredients in a bowl until well combined.
2. Roll into bite-sized balls and chill in the refrigerator before serving.

Nutrition Information:

- Calories: 90
- Protein: 3g
- Carbohydrates: 12g
- Fat: 4g
- Fiber: 2g
- Sugar: 4g
- Portion size: 2 energy bites

Banana Nice Cream

Ingredients:

- 3 ripe bananas, sliced and frozen
- 2 tbsp almond milk (or any plant-based milk)
- 1 tsp vanilla extract

Instructions:

1. Blend frozen bananas, almond milk, and vanilla extract in a high-speed blender until smooth.
2. Serve immediately as soft-serve or freeze for 30 minutes for a firmer texture.

Nutrition Information:

- Calories: 120
- Protein: 1g
- Carbohydrates: 30g
- Fat: 0.5g
- Fiber: 3g
- Sugar: 18g
- Portion size: 1 cup

Vegan Lemon Bars

Ingredients:

For the crust:

- 1 cup almond flour
- 1/4 cup coconut oil, melted
- 2 tbsp maple syrup

For the filling:

- 1 cup cashews, soaked in water for 4 hours and drained
- 1/2 cup lemon juice
- Zest of 1 lemon
- 1/4 cup coconut cream
- 1/4 cup maple syrup

Instructions:

1. Preheat oven to 350°F (175°C). Grease a baking dish.
2. Mix almond flour, melted coconut oil, and maple syrup for the crust. Press into the baking dish and bake for 12-15 minutes, until golden brown. Let cool.
3. Blend soaked cashews, lemon juice, lemon zest, coconut cream, and maple syrup until smooth. Pour over the cooled crust.
4. Refrigerate for at least 4 hours or until set. Cut into bars before serving.

Nutrition Information:

- Calories: 180
- Protein: 4g
- Carbohydrates: 18g
- Fat: 11g
- Fiber: 2g
- Sugar: 10g
- Portion size: 1 bar

Almond Butter Cookies

Ingredients:

- 1 cup almond butter
- 1/2 cup coconut sugar
- 1 flax egg (1 tbsp ground flaxseed + 3 tbsp water)
- 1 tsp vanilla extract
- 1/2 tsp baking soda
- Pinch of salt

Instructions:

1. Preheat oven to 350°F (175°C). Line a baking sheet with parchment paper.
2. In a bowl, mix almond butter, coconut sugar, flax egg, vanilla extract, baking soda, and salt until well combined.

3. Roll dough into tablespoon-sized balls and place on the baking sheet. Flatten each ball with a fork.

4. Bake for 10-12 minutes, until edges are golden brown.

5. Let cool on the baking sheet for 5 minutes before transferring to a wire rack to cool completely.

Nutrition Information:

- Calories: 140
- Protein: 4g
- Carbohydrates: 10g
- Fat: 10g
- Fiber: 2g
- Sugar: 6g
- Portion size: 1 cookie

Chia Seed Chocolate Pudding

Ingredients:

- 1/4 cup chia seeds
- 1 cup almond milk (or any plant-based milk)
- 2 tbsp cocoa powder
- 1 tbsp maple syrup
- 1/2 tsp vanilla extract

Instructions:

1. In a bowl, whisk together chia seeds, almond milk, cocoa powder, maple syrup, and vanilla extract.

2. Let it sit for 5 minutes, then whisk again to prevent clumps.

3. Refrigerate for at least 2 hours or overnight until thickened.

4. Stir well before serving. Add toppings like fresh berries or nuts if desired.

Nutrition Information:

*   Calories: 150
*   Protein: 5g
*   Carbohydrates: 20g
*   Fat: 7g
*   Fiber: 10g
*   Sugar: 6g
*   Portion size: 1/2 cup pudding

Mango Sorbet

Ingredients:

*   2 cups frozen mango chunks
*   1/4 cup coconut milk
*   1 tbsp maple syrup (optional)

Instructions:

1. Blend frozen mango chunks, coconut milk, and maple syrup in a food processor or blender until smooth.
2. Serve immediately for a soft sorbet texture, or freeze for 1-2 hours for a firmer sorbet.

Nutrition Information:

- Calories: 120
- Protein: 1g
- Carbohydrates: 28g
- Fat: 2g
- Fiber: 3g
- Sugar: 24g
- Portion size: 1/2 cup

Vegan Apple Crisp

Ingredients:

- 4 cups sliced apples
- 1 tbsp lemon juice
- 1/2 cup rolled oats
- 1/4 cup almond flour
- 1/4 cup coconut sugar
- 1/4 cup coconut oil, melted

- 1 tsp cinnamon
- Pinch of salt

Instructions:

1. Preheat oven to 350°F (175°C). Grease a baking dish.
2. Toss sliced apples with lemon juice and spread evenly in the baking dish.
3. In a bowl, combine oats, almond flour, coconut sugar, melted coconut oil, cinnamon, and salt until crumbly.
4. Sprinkle oat mixture over the apples.
5. Bake for 30-35 minutes, until apples are tender and topping is golden brown.
6. Serve warm, optionally with a scoop of vegan vanilla ice cream.

Nutrition Information:

- Calories: 220
- Protein: 3g
- Carbohydrates: 32g
- Fat: 10g
- Fiber: 5g
- Sugar: 20g
- Portion size: 1/6 of the crisp

Pistachio Date Balls

Ingredients:

- 1 cup pitted dates
- 1/2 cup shelled pistachios
- 1/4 cup unsweetened shredded coconut
- 1 tbsp cocoa powder
- 1/2 tsp vanilla extract
- Pinch of salt

Instructions:

1. In a food processor, blend dates, pistachios, shredded coconut, cocoa powder, vanilla extract, and salt until mixture forms a sticky dough.
2. Roll into tablespoon-sized balls and place on a plate lined with parchment paper.
3. Optional: Roll balls in extra shredded coconut or cocoa powder.
4. Refrigerate for at least 30 minutes before serving.

Nutrition Information:

- Calories: 120
- Protein: 2g
- Carbohydrates: 20g
- Fat: 5g

- Fiber: 3g
- Sugar: 16g
- Portion size: 2 balls

Blueberry Oat Bars

Ingredients:

- 2 cups rolled oats
- 1 cup blueberries (fresh or frozen)
- 1/2 cup almond butter
- 1/4 cup maple syrup
- 1/4 cup almond milk
- 1 tsp vanilla extract
- Pinch of salt

Instructions:

1. Preheat oven to 350°F (175°C). Grease a baking dish or line with parchment paper.
2. In a bowl, mix rolled oats, blueberries, almond butter, maple syrup, almond milk, vanilla extract, and salt until well combined.
3. Press mixture into the prepared baking dish, ensuring it's evenly spread.
4. Bake for 20-25 minutes, until edges are golden brown.

5. Let cool completely before cutting into bars.

Nutrition Information:

- Calories: 180
- Protein: 5g
- Carbohydrates: 25g
- Fat: 7g
- Fiber: 4g
- Sugar: 10g
- Portion size: 1 bar

Coconut Macaroons

Ingredients:

- 2 cups unsweetened shredded coconut
- 1/2 cup coconut cream
- 1/4 cup maple syrup
- 1 tsp vanilla extract
- Pinch of salt

Instructions:

1. Preheat oven to 325°F (160°C). Line a baking sheet with parchment paper.

2. In a bowl, mix shredded coconut, coconut cream, maple syrup, vanilla extract, and salt until well combined.

3. Scoop tablespoon-sized mounds of the mixture onto the prepared baking sheet.

4. Bake for 20-25 minutes, until edges are golden brown.

5. Let cool on the baking sheet for 10 minutes before transferring to a wire rack to cool completely.

Nutrition Information:

- Calories: 120
- Protein: 1g
- Carbohydrates: 10g
- Fat: 9g
- Fiber: 2g
- Sugar: 7g
- Portion size: 2 macaroons

Vegan Carrot Cake

Ingredients:

- 2 cups grated carrots
- 1 cup almond flour
- 1/2 cup coconut flour
- 1/2 cup coconut sugar

- 1/2 cup unsweetened applesauce

- 1/4 cup coconut oil, melted

- 1/4 cup almond milk

- 1 tsp baking powder

- 1 tsp baking soda

- 1 tsp cinnamon

- 1/2 tsp nutmeg

- 1/4 tsp salt

- 1/2 cup chopped walnuts (optional)

- Vegan cream cheese frosting (optional)

Instructions:

1. Preheat oven to 350°F (175°C). Grease a cake pan or line with parchment paper.

2. In a large bowl, combine grated carrots, almond flour, coconut flour, coconut sugar, applesauce, melted coconut oil, almond milk, baking powder, baking soda, cinnamon, nutmeg, and salt. Mix until well combined.

3. Fold in chopped walnuts if using.

4. Pour batter into the prepared cake pan and spread evenly.

5. Bake for 30-35 minutes, until a toothpick inserted into the center comes out clean.

6. Let cool completely before frosting with vegan cream cheese frosting if desired.

Nutrition Information:

- Calories: 250
- Protein: 5g
- Carbohydrates: 30g
- Fat: 13g
- Fiber: 5g
- Sugar: 15g
- Portion size: 1/12 of cake

Peanut Butter Chocolate Chip Blondies

Ingredients:

- 1 cup creamy peanut butter
- 1/2 cup coconut sugar
- 1/4 cup maple syrup
- 1/4 cup almond milk
- 1 tsp vanilla extract
- 1 cup oat flour
- 1/2 tsp baking soda
- 1/2 cup dairy-free chocolate chips

Instructions:

1. Preheat oven to 350°F (175°C). Grease a baking dish or line with parchment paper.

2. In a bowl, mix peanut butter, coconut sugar, maple syrup, almond milk, and vanilla extract until smooth.

3. Add oat flour and baking soda, mixing until well combined.

4. Fold in chocolate chips.

5. Spread batter evenly into the prepared baking dish.

6. Bake for 20-25 minutes, until edges are golden brown and a toothpick inserted into the center comes out clean.

7. Let cool completely before cutting into squares.

Nutrition Information:

- Calories: 200
- Protein: 6g
- Carbohydrates: 20g
- Fat: 12g
- Fiber: 2g
- Sugar: 10g
- Portion size: 1 blondie

Raspberry Almond Thumbprint Cookies

Ingredients:

- 1 cup almond flour
- 1/4 cup coconut oil, melted
- 1/4 cup maple syrup

- 1/2 tsp almond extract
- Raspberry jam (or any fruit jam of choice)

Instructions:

1. Preheat oven to 350°F (175°C). Line a baking sheet with parchment paper.
2. In a bowl, mix almond flour, melted coconut oil, maple syrup, and almond extract until dough forms.
3. Roll dough into tablespoon-sized balls and place on the prepared baking sheet.
4. Make an indentation in the center of each cookie with your thumb or the back of a spoon.
5. Spoon a small amount of raspberry jam into each indentation.
6. Bake for 10-12 minutes, until cookies are golden brown.
7. Let cool on the baking sheet for 5 minutes before transferring to a wire rack to cool completely.

Nutrition Information:

- Calories: 150
- Protein: 3g
- Carbohydrates: 12g
- Fat: 10g
- Fiber: 2g

- Sugar: 7g
- Portion size: 2 cookies

Chapter 7: Smoothies

Smoothies are a refreshing and nutritious way to start your day or refuel after a workout. Packed with vitamins, minerals, and antioxidants, these smoothie recipes are designed to support your health and provide a delicious treat. Whether you're looking for a green detox option or a fruity indulgence, there's a smoothie here to suit every taste and dietary preference.

Green Detox Smoothie

Ingredients:

- 1 cup spinach
- 1/2 cucumber, peeled and sliced
- 1 celery stalk, chopped
- 1/2 green apple, cored and chopped
- Juice of 1/2 lemon
- 1 cup coconut water
- Ice cubes (optional)

Instructions:

1. Place all ingredients in a blender.
2. Blend until smooth.
3. Pour into a glass and serve immediately.

Nutrition Information (per serving):

- Calories: 80
- Protein: 2g
- Carbohydrates: 18g
- Fat: 0.5g
- Fiber: 4g
- Sugar: 10g
- Portion Size: 1 smoothie

Berry Blast Smoothie

Ingredients:

- 1 cup mixed berries (strawberries, blueberries, raspberries)
- 1/2 banana
- 1/2 cup plain Greek yogurt (or dairy-free yogurt)
- 1 tbsp honey or maple syrup (optional)
- 1/2 cup almond milk (or any milk of choice)
- Ice cubes (optional)

Instructions:

1. Combine all ingredients in a blender.
2. Blend until smooth.
3. Pour into a glass and enjoy!

Nutrition Information (per serving):

- Calories: 150
- Protein: 6g
- Carbohydrates: 30g
- Fat: 2g
- Fiber: 5g
- Sugar: 20g
- Portion Size: 1 smoothie

Mango Turmeric Smoothie

Ingredients:

- 1 cup chopped mango
- 1/2 banana
- 1/2 tsp turmeric powder
- 1/2 tsp fresh ginger, grated
- 1 cup coconut water or almond milk
- Ice cubes (optional)

Instructions:

1. Combine all ingredients in a blender.
2. Blend until smooth.
3. Serve immediately.

Nutrition Information (per serving):

- Calories: 140
- Protein: 2g
- Carbohydrates: 32g
- Fat: 1g
- Fiber: 4g
- Sugar: 25g
- Portion Size: 1 smoothie

Spinach Pineapple Smoothie

Ingredients:

- 1 cup fresh spinach
- 1 cup chopped pineapple
- 1/2 banana
- 1/2 cup plain Greek yogurt (or dairy-free yogurt)
- 1/2 cup coconut water or pineapple juice
- Ice cubes (optional)

Instructions:

1. Place all ingredients in a blender.
2. Blend until smooth.
3. Pour into a glass and enjoy!

Nutrition Information (per serving):

- Calories: 160
- Protein: 6g
- Carbohydrates: 35g
- Fat: 1g
- Fiber: 4g
- Sugar: 25g
- Portion Size: 1 smoothie

Chocolate Peanut Butter Smoothie

Ingredients:

- 1 banana
- 1 tbsp cocoa powder
- 1 tbsp natural peanut butter
- 1 cup almond milk (or any milk of choice)
- 1 tbsp honey or maple syrup (optional)
- Ice cubes (optional)

Instructions:

1. Combine all ingredients in a blender.
2. Blend until smooth and creamy.
3. Pour into a glass and serve immediately.

Nutrition Information (per serving):

- Calories: 250

- Protein: 7g

- Carbohydrates: 36g

- Fat: 10g

- Fiber: 5g

- Sugar: 20g

- Portion Size: 1 smoothie

Kale Banana Smoothie

Ingredients:

- 1 cup chopped kale leaves

- 1 banana

- 1/2 cup plain Greek yogurt (or dairy-free yogurt)

- 1 tbsp chia seeds

- 1 tbsp honey or maple syrup (optional)

- 1 cup almond milk (or any milk of choice)

- Ice cubes (optional)

Instructions:

1. Place all ingredients in a blender.

2. Blend until smooth.

3. Pour into a glass and enjoy!

Nutrition Information (per serving):

- Calories: 180
- Protein: 9g
- Carbohydrates: 32g
- Fat: 4g
- Fiber: 6g
- Sugar: 18g
- Portion Size: 1 smoothie

Tropical Mango Smoothie

Ingredients:

- 1 cup chopped mango
- 1/2 cup chopped pineapple
- 1/2 banana
- 1/2 cup coconut water or pineapple juice
- 1/4 cup Greek yogurt (or dairy-free yogurt)
- Ice cubes (optional)

Instructions:

1. Combine all ingredients in a blender.
2. Blend until smooth.
3. Pour into a glass and serve immediately.

Nutrition Information (per serving):

- Calories: 180
- Protein: 5g
- Carbohydrates: 40g
- Fat: 1g
- Fiber: 4g
- Sugar: 30g
- Portion Size: 1 smoothie

Blueberry Almond Butter Smoothie

Ingredients:

- 1 cup blueberries
- 1 banana
- 2 tbsp almond butter
- 1 cup almond milk (or any milk of choice)
- 1 tbsp honey or maple syrup (optional)
- Ice cubes (optional)

Instructions:

1. Place all ingredients in a blender.
2. Blend until smooth.
3. Pour into a glass and enjoy!

Nutrition Information (per serving):

- Calories: 280
- Protein: 7g
- Carbohydrates: 40g
- Fat: 12g
- Fiber: 8g
- Sugar: 25g
- Portion Size: 1 smoothie

Beetroot Berry Smoothie

Ingredients:

- 1/2 cup cooked and peeled beetroot
- 1/2 cup mixed berries (strawberries, raspberries, blueberries)
- 1/2 banana
- 1 cup almond milk (or any milk of choice)
- 1 tbsp honey or maple syrup (optional)
- Ice cubes (optional)

Instructions:

1. Combine all ingredients in a blender.
2. Blend until smooth.
3. Serve immediately.

Nutrition Information (per serving):

- Calories: 160
- Protein: 3g
- Carbohydrates: 35g
- Fat: 2g
- Fiber: 7g
- Sugar: 25g
- Portion Size: 1 smoothie

Avocado Spinach Smoothie

Ingredients:

- 1/2 ripe avocado
- 1 cup fresh spinach
- 1/2 banana
- Juice of 1/2 lime
- 1 cup coconut water or almond milk
- Ice cubes (optional)

Instructions:

1. Place all ingredients in a blender.
2. Blend until smooth.
3. Pour into a glass and enjoy!

Nutrition Information (per serving):

- Calories: 200
- Protein: 4g
- Carbohydrates: 25g
- Fat: 11g
- Fiber: 7g
- Sugar: 10g
- Portion Size: 1 smoothie

Chai Spiced Smoothie

Ingredients:

- 1/2 cup brewed chai tea, chilled
- 1/2 cup plain Greek yogurt (or dairy-free yogurt)
- 1/2 banana
- 1/2 tsp ground cinnamon
- 1/4 tsp ground ginger
- 1/4 tsp ground cardamom
- 1 tbsp honey or maple syrup (optional)
- Ice cubes (optional)

Instructions:

1. Combine all ingredients in a blender.
2. Blend until smooth.

3. Pour into a glass and serve immediately.

Nutrition Information (per serving):

- Calories: 130
- Protein: 8g
- Carbohydrates: 25g
- Fat: 1g
- Fiber: 2g
- Sugar: 18g
- Portion Size: 1 smoothie

Pineapple Coconut Smoothie

Ingredients:

- 1 cup chopped pineapple
- 1/2 cup coconut milk
- 1/2 banana
- 1/4 cup shredded coconut (unsweetened)
- 1 tbsp honey or maple syrup (optional)
- Ice cubes (optional)

Instructions:

1. Place all ingredients in a blender.
2. Blend until smooth.

3. Pour into a glass and enjoy!

Nutrition Information (per serving):

- Calories: 220
- Protein: 2g
- Carbohydrates: 35g
- Fat: 9g
- Fiber: 3g
- Sugar: 25g
- Portion Size: 1 smoothie

Raspberry Beet Smoothie

Ingredients:

- 1/2 cup cooked and peeled beetroot
- 1/2 cup raspberries
- 1/2 banana
- 1/2 cup almond milk (or any milk of choice)
- 1 tbsp honey or maple syrup (optional)
- Ice cubes (optional)

Instructions:

1. Combine all ingredients in a blender.
2. Blend until smooth.

3. Serve immediately.

Nutrition Information (per serving):

- Calories: 160
- Protein: 3g
- Carbohydrates: 35g
- Fat: 2g
- Fiber: 7g
- Sugar: 20g
- Portion Size: 1 smoothie

Orange Carrot Ginger Smoothie

Ingredients:

- 1 orange, peeled and segmented
- 1 carrot, peeled and chopped
- 1/2 inch piece of fresh ginger, grated
- 1/2 cup Greek yogurt (or dairy-free yogurt)
- 1/2 cup orange juice
- Ice cubes (optional)

Instructions:

1. Place all ingredients in a blender.
2. Blend until smooth.

3. Pour into a glass and serve immediately.

Nutrition Information (per serving):

- Calories: 150
- Protein: 6g
- Carbohydrates: 30g
- Fat: 1g
- Fiber: 4g
- Sugar: 22g
- Portion Size: 1 smoothie

Papaya Lime Smoothie

Ingredients:

- 1 cup chopped papaya
- Juice of 1 lime
- 1/2 banana
- 1/2 cup coconut water or almond milk
- 1 tbsp honey or maple syrup (optional)
- Ice cubes (optional)

Instructions:

1. Combine all ingredients in a blender.
2. Blend until smooth.

3. Pour into a glass and enjoy!

Nutrition Information (per serving):

- Calories: 140
- Protein: 2g
- Carbohydrates: 30g
- Fat: 1g
- Fiber: 3g
- Sugar: 20g
- Portion Size: 1 smoothie

CONCLUSION

Congratulations on completing your journey through the "Prediabetes Meal Planning Cookbook for Vegetarians and Vegans"! This cookbook has been crafted with your health and well-being in mind, offering a wealth of delicious and nutritious recipes tailored specifically for managing prediabetes through vegetarian and vegan diets.

Throughout this book, you've discovered the power of plant-based foods in stabilizing blood sugar levels and promoting overall health. From hearty breakfasts to satisfying dinners, from energizing smoothies to guilt-free desserts, each recipe has been designed not only to tantalize your taste buds but also to support your journey towards better health.

By embracing a diet rich in fruits, vegetables, whole grains, legumes, nuts, and seeds, you've taken proactive steps towards managing your prediabetes and improving your quality of life. The 30-day meal plan has provided structure and convenience, helping you navigate your dietary choices with ease.

Remember, this cookbook is not just a collection of recipes; it's a tool to empower you in your daily food choices. Whether you're new to vegetarianism or veganism or have been practicing for years, the variety of recipes ensures there's something delightful for every palate and occasion.

As you move forward, continue to experiment with these recipes, personalize them to suit your tastes, and explore the vast array of plant-based ingredients available to you. Stay mindful of portion sizes, listen to your body's cues, and maintain regular physical activity to complement your dietary efforts.

Lastly, use the knowledge and inspiration gained from this cookbook to foster a sustainable and enjoyable approach to eating well with prediabetes. Here's to your health, happiness, and a future filled with vibrant meals that nourish both body and soul.

Thank you for choosing this cookbook as your guide. May your journey towards managing prediabetes be fulfilling, flavorful, and full of vitality!